FAMILY TIES

FAMILY TIES

AVERY NIGHTINGALE

CONTENTS

CHAPTER 1

Introduction

S uch trends highlight the importance of interdisciplinary action for policies that will offer different means of care and assistance to the elderly, while simultaneously respecting their dignity, autonomy, and personal resources. In this context, it is important for countries to understand social structures and living arrangements that can potentially influence public and community policies, where older adults and their descendants can then share and benefit from their knowledge, experiences, and care for each other. With the complexity of aging processes and the influence of diversity in living arrangements of families worldwide, national, regional, and local efforts should recognize the demographic, economic, and cultural dimensions of this population phenomenon and the family support system.

With advances in healthcare, healthy lifestyle choices, and the rising standards of living, most of today's people will live longer than previous generations did. As a result of this trend, the population is aging in many countries worldwide. For example, currently 8.3% of the world's population is over 65 years of age, and this percentage is projected to increase to 25.5% by the year 2050. As people start living longer, increasing numbers of individuals in this age group will experience symptoms of cognitive decline and disease, which is estimated to reach as high as 16 million worldwide by that time. As a result of this trend, it is often said that families will have four generations alive in their lifetime, including children, parents, and grandparents.

CHAPTER 2

Importance of Family Bonds

As for extended families, the elders who have reached old age will be taken care of by the younger generation. This is because as human beings age, their bodily abilities will become weak and fragile, and as they age further, the elders will not be able to look after the members of their family themselves. Therefore, members of their family will take it upon themselves to look after the elders, like the elders themselves had looked after them when they were younger. Furthermore, this kind of relationship creates a sense of unity and mutual respect. As such, this relationship dissipates with the death of the previous generations in the family unit, and the feelings of love and respect towards the predecessors are carried down from the elders to the youngest among the family members.

In general, family ties are the relationships that exist in different types of families, such as nuclear family members or extended family members. These kinds of family ties are important in helping to establish a family foundation based on respect, support, and love. In a nuclear family, good parent-child relationships are very important in helping to educate their children. In addition, relationships with each other can also educate the children in the supervision of the elderly. When these good relations are maintained, parents can guide their children up to adulthood, even when the children have their own families in the future.

CHAPTER 3

Understanding Generational Differences

As we have already reflected in the first part of our consideration "Within the family," the connection between generations is not always so linear. Changes in society, in consumption habits, in economic problems, in experience, all contribute to generating changes and conflicts. How to understand these big differences between parents and children? Can we do something to minimize the negative effects of these influences or simply control the different sources so that they do not break or end our good family harmony? One of the conflicts that has always existed between generations is the difference in customs. For instance, when we see the behavior of fishermen in fisherpeople's family, we find practices and customs that are very different from ours. How not to be curious about what we see, hear, and feel associated with such different cultural backgrounds that we have lived? With this observation, we must also recognize that this difference, as much as it may catch our attention, is a natural process from a society.

There really is no other explanation for the criticism you hear coming from different generations: "Why do they do that?" or "When I was their age, I did this"? Most families at some point in time find themselves wondering how cultural differences and practices affect the child-rearing process. How much are these differences the result of family values and norms that came from traditions? Have we ever stopped to ask ourselves about the origin of prejudices or fear of the unknown? Never have we ever stopped to reflect on other types of customs and traditions. How to deal with this giant that is within our homes called the generation gap?

CHAPTER 4

Communication Strategies

It is in initial placement that trust is built, and this trust between professionals, family, and carers will be a key indicator and predictor of where the child will be placed. Social services must continually support the contact between the extended family as well as the birth family if appropriate. Over time, the role that grandparents play will become invaluable, and the bond that the carer shared with grandparents would reflect the carer's understanding of this network in the eyes of the professional. Reassurances would need to be given in that the birth family and grandparents would be respected and encouraged to take an active role with the children. Social services will have to overcome previous distrust of agencies and professionals and ensure that the concerns and wants of these carers are met, while also understanding that their reluctance has its foundations in fear.

Grandparents and extended family are particularly important for foster families and should be nurtured. Foster carers need to plan time for grandparents and extended family to build a relationship with their grandchild. Without this support, foster families may feel that they are on their own in the foster caring role. Social services should also consider the family's request for information when possible about their grandchild. If at all possible, they should include the family when inviting parents to meeting or sharing information. Good practice would include prioritizing grandparents on the "chain of information." It is largely through these local family networks that foster relationships are nurtured and built upon. Social services need to be mindful that not all foster carers understand family network systems, especially if their network of support is comprised of professionals.

CHAPTER 5

Building Trust and Respect

To start, there must be trust that the care we give to those who have provided such service to us was or will be appreciated or reciprocated. There must be respect for what those who were young, bright, and full of visions for the future in days past have to offer or share. When those bonds exist in family relationships, the act of caregiving transitions into an act of memory making and the act of receiving care becomes a tangible representation of respect and love toward a family elder while enabling and encouraging the sharing of stories and wisdom.

Respect is something built and shared through our everyday lives. It provides the niche for a family to truly bond with one another. When we are all truly valued for who we are, we gain happiness, health, and a wealth of support from the bonds that we build. Where trust and respect lay solid, all remaining foundations of family truly flourish.

Trust comes hand in hand with making memories and spending time. It also comes with teaching and being taught truth. This trust becomes increasingly important as we rely on each other to provide care and support for one another.

For any relationship, trust and respect are vital. But they also evolve and strengthen over time. It doesn't take much prompting from television or a good read to make most people want to cherish memories and spend time, even more time, with their loved ones. It doesn't take more than a little social media to make many people feel like their families could be closer. And as our children grow into the many seasons of their lives, we'll find many opportunities, or excuses, for truly being together as a family.

CHAPTER 6

Nurturing Emotional Connections

Bonding and emotional connections can be nurtured when every member respects the other, when you consistently care for each other, when you cater to your relationship, when members truly involve themselves in each other's lives, when there is freedom to talk, when you spend time with one another, when you always support one another, when you have genuine respect for the other person's struggle, when you are transparent, doing things together, and when you avoid telling and doing negative things about one another. You may decide to have family activities at least twice a year. It would give you an opportunity to bond more deeply. In such occasions, activities such as eating together, cooking, sharing stories of your childhood, sharing love letters to the children, telling spiritual stories, doing sacred things together, going to a park, playing games, and many other activities that the family members love to do where all participate.

Bonding is important for the family as it brings members closer to one another, provides members with a sense of security, and gives them an opportunity to share the happy and unhappy moments of each other's lives. Bonding or building connections with family members is an emotional process. This requires expressing natural love, being there for family members, and cheering each other's achievements. Everyone needs a good bond with their family members. Being truly connected becomes hard when family ties weaken due to several reasons, such as when both parents go to work, estrangement (no longer involved in a relationship or attending social functions), broken families, emotional blackmail, using money to dominate, guilt, and many other reasons. However, bonding or connection can be strengthened with some attention and consciousness.

CHAPTER 7

Sharing Family Traditions

Within the fabric of celebrations like Christmas are the cherished traditions that bind families, young and old, to one another. The keyboards of computers buzz with the renewal of family connections built over the year through packages and bags of sweets and treats sent to loved ones. Traditions are the love that wrap the world and propel it into the future. They are how our societies reflect and strengthen the bonds, cultures, and foundations of love and faith we have for one another.

"The planning begins months in advance, making sure there is the correct equipment for the cookie baking, the correct recipe cards, the right variety of nuts, chocolate, powdered sugars, and colored jells. Then the actual shopping at the store."

Perhaps the most common of rituals during the holiday season is the practice of baking or cooking a special recipe handed down through the generations. Children look forward to the first bite of sweets like the hallmark sugar cookie, handed down through the generations and prepared with love and history. Men and women plan these rituals all year, which tie them to the memorable moments of the past. A woman from New Jersey recalls a cherished tradition with her Aunt Kitty Bailey during the Christmas season.

CHAPTER 8

Creating Meaningful Memories

That tangible thing in my hands - my joy - becomes something I could look at whenever I need to. I know it will evoke a smile. The kids might flip through it and remember their childhood. I get warm fuzzies from the anticipation of their memories about the good times we've had. Sometimes they've even asked questions about vacations and things we did together. It's a way of bringing our experiences into the present.

To get to this point in my life, I've learned that I need to keep family time at the top of my priority list. I want my kids to look back on their days and realize that we were present with each other. We didn't always take everyday experiences too seriously, but we made them worthwhile. We made them joyous. We tried to create joy together. Photographs are a way of immortalizing a moment, and there have been moments that I wanted to last forever. I wanted to grasp them and refuse to let them go. But once they're captured, they're preserved for always in my favorite photo album. I carefully tape or glue them in, knowing that without this act, they might get lost or ruined.

The best part about memories is making them. If you're not careful, you can go through your whole day without stopping to make a memory. I've realized that memories of family time aren't always big events. It can be the simple things like making a meal together, practicing soccer drills in the backyard, or going for a bike ride. It's those "everyday" moments that mean so much. They matter.

CHAPTER 9

Balancing Independence and Dependence

Balance between dependence and independence is inextricably interwoven with the capacity of members to communicate and negotiate conflict as well as navigate distance, speed, and information needs among and between family groups. Issues of distance or attachment of geographical units spanning distance are also hampered/bolstered by available coping resources (physical and social) and information/referral networks to deal with everyday problems and crises. The merger of caring needs with appropriate remedies and the nature of this interaction distinguishes grandparent caregiving from grandparent investments in their grandchildren. Early child development serves as the most obtainable example of the link between dependence, independence, and reintegration on care and socialization.

From childhood through adolescence, the journey toward self-sufficiency introduces children to independent life. Developmental achievement of autonomy, independence, and self-sufficiency is a familiar paradigm applied in many areas, notably the field of psychology. Such notions have also been applied in family scholarship from several perspectives, including the family life cycle and systems theory. Intrapsychic, individual, and family system issues also affect this journey into adulthood and the nuclear family lifestyle. This chapter, however, argues that the attainment of independence begins less visionary than is usually assumed. Three specific family functions – care, mediation, and socialization – supported a new independence and maturity that was an outgrowth of earlier behavior modes and expectations.

CHAPTER 10

Supporting Aging Family Members

The best gift for an aging relative can be our love and joy, and to diligently care for them as they age. Our love flows from our experiences and memories of being together doing things that are fun; the essence of this fun will die out if it's limited to a few moments a year. Furthermore, these fun activities break down to conversing, doing various chores around the house, discussing goals and fears, and the sense of security in taking time together. Communication, care, and interesting activities strengthen family connections, and our elderly realize their lives are important, even in physical decline. By intermingling concerns and looking out for one another - sharing feelings of burdens or simple chores around the house - our elderly gain a sense of belonging. Encouraging them to be more active and integrated limits their loneliness or feelings of despair. As we age, good-quality time spent with family members becomes imperative to maintain health and wellness; healthy relationships ward off anxiety, depression, and debilitating illnesses that wear down the human spirit.

The past century has witnessed a dramatic increase in the average human lifespan due in part to advances in medicine, infrastructure, and a variety of societal changes that have contributed to our increased understanding of wellness and overall well-being. Being able to share the joys and challenges with parents, grandparents, or extended family members in the various stages of becoming older is a real privilege. No matter how many years separate one generation from the next, the love and connection that exists is a testimonial to the unique time spent together. Lifelong family relationships are indispensable for children's well-being and growth, which extends the human life cycle, promoting a sense of purpose and meaning in life. Therefore, it's important to cultivate family connections, love, and mutual assistance among younger and older family members.

CHAPTER 11

Fostering Intergenerational Relationships

It is certainly desirable, from a traditional perspective, that families be as cohesive as possible. But it may be more productive to consider families not as discrete entities with specific boundaries but as a series of relationships that stand on their own feet and operate on their own merits. Interactions within extended families keep the elders as well as the young from being isolated. More elders today are living in isolation from their traditional hosts, who are preoccupied with fulfilling honorific rites as well meeting the demands of a consuming modern lifestyle.

One of the best ways to get "more life" out of the life you have left is to build and nurture relationships across the ages. The oldest members of our society can draw energy and revitalization from contact with younger generations. They can pass down knowledge, tradition, and values, quickly and effectively. The young, in turn, can learn to understand and tolerate the foibles of their elders; to appreciate their collective experiences, customs, and values; and to discern and navigate a path through the complexities of life. Many organizations are helping to link people of different ages around common interests. Dozens of "senior aid programs" link seniors with a need to young adults who fill these needs, under the sponsorship of organizations or agencies that coordinate efforts of the youth involved. For example, perhaps an elder museum-goer would like to use her free pass more often, but she does not have a driver's license. She can give her free pass to a young girl, who is able to get there herself, and they can meet inside the museum to tour together. Seniors get the assistance and company they need, and the young adult gets a social experience, cultural exposure, and a little fun on the side.

CHAPTER 12

Strengthening Sibling Bonds

The following reflections, shared memories, and lessons learned may be useful to brothers and sisters, cousins, nephews, and nieces with similar dual attachments to their siblings and to their own selves. We posit that these hybrid familial and personal connections interact to strengthen each other. Based on these dialectical perspectives, this chapter explores the importance of strong sibling and genetic connections to aging well. We describe unique and overlapping strengths of our "sib-pair" and twin relationships and show the benefits we have derived from them through the years. We submit that the unique dynamics of sibling and genetic alliances across life are important to comprehend, celebrate, and engage in, especially in times of adversity. Then, a fundamental discussion of individual multigenerational sibling ideals as both empirical and ethical perspectives complements practical examples of using our each ability. Collectively, these case studies enable us to flourish across time on personal, family, and cultural levels by focusing on the broader view of identity response, editorial reflections on the significance of our sib-pair identity, in order to attain new life goals.

My siblings and I continue to share numerous family stories, reminiscences, and inside jokes. We share fun and laughs through our "This Is Your Life" board game when we answer questions based on information about each other. We sing the songs our father taught us when he bounced us on his knees. We visit and tease each other. We turn to each other for sympathy and comfort. We go and grow out to lunch and dinner together. In getting to know each other not only as brothers but also as human souls, we have found much to like and admire in each other. Our family cloak, carefully and lovingly woven through the years, allows us to sit comfortably in each other's company, despite our differing lives. Four brothers, three sisters, and I have survived into our older age and have managed to stay close through occasional get-togethers, phone calls, text messages, birthdays, anniversaries, and frequent emails. Since my waking moments are precious, I've chosen to spend more of them with the people who have always cheered me on, volunteers at my fundraisers, and contributed to my greatest childhood happiness: my brothers and sisters. With our aging parents at the center of family activities, growing up together recognized common bonds woven in the core of our beings, threads that could never be removed - threads of shared struggles, joys, and growth, that tied us to our sibling community. Corroborating, celebrating, and absorbing these connections from generations of family ties across time brought emotional and spiritual connectedness that helped us create and sustain both lasting and novel relationships between and among our genes and generations - relationships we know now to be central to our resilience as we grow older.

Friends say it must have been difficult growing up on a farm with nine brothers and sisters, but I remember it differently. I remember it as constant noise, constant activity, and constant playmates. I remember that I was never bored and never lonely. I remember that there was always someone to talk to, someone to share stories or secrets with, someone to play with or to play a trick on. I remember fun and camaraderie. I don't remember the work, the farming, the poverty, or the parents' problems.

CHAPTER 13

Grandparent-Grandchild Relationships

Grandparents care for and transmit cultural customs and information to grandchildren. In turn, grandchildren care for the well-being of their grandparents. This reciprocal relationship is important. As the age gap between grandparents and their grandchild increases, different and stronger channels of communication emerge between generations. The grandparent-grandparent relationship becomes particularly important when the grandchild is raised by a single mother. It is widely believed in many societies that multigenerational co-residence and contact between grandparents, grandchildren, and their parents are important for the development of values and socialization. For example, the findings reveal that young people grow in a family with a grandparent who assumes an educative role that fosters interaction. It also reveals that, on the contrary, the lack of physical contact between the grandparents and the grandchildren often affects the educational participation of the parents and the difficult children and creates dissatisfaction and emotional problems in both groups.

One of the most primary relationships that exists in the family is the bond between grandparents and grandchildren. With longer and healthier lives, both the numbers and presence of grandparents are increasing. Some children are fortunate to have their grandparents. The structure of the grandparent-grandchild relationship is changing because of demographic changes. For example, the birth rate is declining. As a result, grandparents have fewer grandchildren to share their time, love, wisdom, and resources with. And with increased life expectancy, each person is living longer. This implies that both adult children and grandchildren have longer lives. Consequently, there might be a large age gap between grandparents and their younger grandchild. These grandparents have sufficient time to accumulate wealth and/or assets and resources to invest in the education of their grandchildren. For these reasons also, the number of multigenerational households is increasing, intergenerational transfer by grandparents is becoming relatively more important, and both generations perceive the family as a major force in transferring values.

CHAPTER 14

Parent-Child Relationships

That the parent-child relationship does influence thoughts and behaviors, and that individuals' individualization is characterized by both positive and negative features. These various ideas are especially important, as they demonstrate that even this period of adjustment is seen as an opportunity for more personal growth and potential to continue the learning process. By considering their work burden as only one part of both professional and family life, the decision to keep children close also means that this future generation of older adults takes care of their own aging parent. In order for parents to feel that they and their children mutually contribute to the well-being of one another in a meaningful way and that family exchange is two-way, at the same time today's adult children continue beyond age 40 to have a relationship of shared support with their parents.

The parent-child relationship and adult well-being have been extensively studied by sociologists and demographers because of its staying power and implications for such areas as social inequality and economic productivity. Establishing and maintaining good relationships for parents and their children is a notion that has been around for centuries, but a point where it has been stressed by baby boomers and their like-minded predecessors is when children have left home and established their own independent lives. Recent scholars of a more optimistic, risk-taking nature talk about the possibilities of increased autonomy between parents and children, while other studies note that there will naturally be higher levels of integrity and happiness from living independent lives.

CHAPTER 15

Extended Family Connections

In a neighborhood with few options for social engagement, the center is typically packed. "The seniors really look forward to NPC Thursday afternoons," says Valerie Padilla, the NPC family services coordinator there. At first, younger family members—some visiting their elders at the center for the first time in years—predominated at extended family events, but now they are steadily attracting seniors' neighbors as well.

Then, two years ago, the center, a Neighborhood Partners in Care (NPC) project, began organizing an extended family program. The program focuses on building social connections for seniors by not only helping them, but also by engaging family members and others whose social support may be essential to their health and well-being.

Maria Torres has lived in the same East Los Angeles house for 45 years, and she and her family are deeply rooted in the community. Her son and daughters still live nearby, and she is a frequent visitor to the neighborhood senior center. But even with so many family members nearby, at 82 Torres has sometimes felt isolated and lonely, amid a sea of activities.

CHAPTER 16

Embracing Diversity and Inclusion

We suggest this, with the firm belief that the space occupied by the past is no less important than the future that we propose to build. Recalling this "mined" space, extracting the most convincing notions from it and exploiting them in order to steady and guide us can be an invaluable resource. When evaluating the past, we should adopt the most inclusive and diverse perspective possible, which minimizes misunderstandings. We should take advantage of the experience and ability of social scientists and scientists working in all fields to provide relevant information and explain clearly issues surrounding the present reality.

Throughout 2020, the global pandemic that has shaken the world has aggravated and continues to do so a great many controversies and challenges whose solutions need time in order to be clearly defined and accepted and implemented. Besides the regrettable deaths caused by the pandemic, large numbers of people have lost their jobs and businesses have been forced to close, with many more millions of people fearing similar collapses to occur. In attempting to face and solve the unprecedented disturbances and crises on the scale of those demonstrated in 2020, we suggest to those responsible for making decisions and proposing, recommending, and putting into practice such decisions that in doing so they do everything possible to embody, in their attempts to do so, our shared story of our past, thus taking maximum advantage of such an invaluable resource.

Overcoming Generational Stereotypes

More remote emotional signaling between this generation of young people and their elders can be confused by both with rejection of each other (and the lengthening of life; people in developed countries are now living 30 years longer than they did just 100 years ago) holding to such stereotypes for a lifetime. After the early adolescent period, the stereotypes don't remain constant, but they rarely change in response to new stimuli. With persistence, these attitudes become more institutionalized and difficult to remove. Younger people are then forced to live their adult lives and create young citizens based on these stereotypes, which will not show major change for a lifetime. Just as the critical event can gain increased influence in the absence of challenge, the same is true for positive experiences.

Younger people show the same feelings except in reverse. Why is such an early-age critical event so influential? Early adolescence is a tumultuous time involving – among other things – a "self-inflicted" child-identity change and fewer overtures of love and admiration from adults. Teens struggle with both identity and morality; and this period of adjustment is naturally traumatic in order to help the teen learn to adapt to a greater number of social situations – which produces a more moral outcome.

1) Do you mind when teenagers ignore you? 2) Do you think young people nowadays are only interested in themselves?

My research indicates that there are ways to expedite a similar respect among generations. Each generation has negative stereotypes of all others, typically the result of a critical event that occurred when they were in early adolescence (age 11-13). Older people also usually answer yes to one or both of the following questions:

How do we know when it's time to let go of the myths that prevent us from seeing the rich complexity of these older people? Personal relationships are one way that younger generations can come to know and respect older generations. Young people are always looking for someone who makes them feel respected, and when respected, tend to respect in return. Throughout history, it has been the case that respect for beliefs, even when completely different, achieves things and preserves relationships; and this is much more valuable during tough times when we often depend on each other.

CHAPTER 18

Managing Family Dynamics

Remember that this exercise tests both the listeners and the speakers; if one member hogs the time, others should voice their concerns after this announcement, "Your cogent points are duly noted. I'd like to hear from some other voices which have yet to contribute." Families must redefine the work ethic and its management processes to align personal strengths and interests with family goals. This means having conversations with children about their future, dreams, hobbies and personal goals. Teach them to define their "missions and visions" as well as cultivating your firm understanding of who they are. Creating a common mission with shared objectives is crucial in maintaining focus and sustaining the essential management systems. Also virtually eliminate "workaholic family reimbursement."

Empower everyone to contribute. Start by engaging everyone in a family communication exercise without discussing it first. Begin by giving everyone an opportunity to talk uninterrupted and without being asked questions. It's a practice for the family leader or leader-to-be to sit quietly and listen, but it's also essential for everyone to practice speaking honestly and openly, in a safe environment where there can never be any recriminations. Family czars must cultivate a consulting system, presenting their subject to the group, engaging them in discussion and finally making decisions with their input.

CHAPTER 19

Coping with Loss and Grief

The manuscript discusses how during this time Casey, Elizabeth, and their sisters gained firsthand experience with older relatives with Alzheimer's disease, mobility problems, and other limitations due to advancing age. That knowledge and the close bonds between the students and their older relatives influenced their consideration of college locations, college and graduate major selection, future educational and occupational goals, and family-related career decisions. In addition, the knowledge and caregiving experiences affected their relationships with their roommates, romantic partners, bodies, and college transitions.

Elizabeth's mother is Kat, Casey's best friend in third grade, and after her father divorced her mother when she was seven, Kat and Elizabeth maintained a close relationship with Casey and her family. Casey and Elizabeth are especially close to one another's siblings and parents and describe themselves as relatives more than as friends. The closest grandparent to die was Alyson, Elizabeth's paternal grandmother, who had been very close to Casey during her childhood and frequently visited Elizabeth and her other grandchildren in her later years. Toward the end of high school, Elizabeth was also hospitalized with an eating disorder, and Kat did not leave her side during Elizabeth's weeks in the hospital. Over ten years, from Casey's seventh-grade year to Elizabeth's first year in college, the two girls and their sisters spent an increasing amount of time with their grandparents, often in the family's living room.

Casey and Henry were close to both their maternal and paternal grandparents, and when Casey started college in 2005, all but one of those grandparents was living. Henry, Casey's cousin, was a few years older than Casey but started college at the same time. Casey and Henry were very close when they were young, and Henry described Casey as his best friend and his "sister from different parents." Casey and Henry's college experiences were very different, in part because of their parents' and families' different approaches to dealing with grief and their grandparents' deaths. I draw on actual quotes from Casey, her family, her grandmother's diary, and Henry to illustrate how family relationships - employment, income, household size, and death of close family members - affect college students' mental health and can also influence their occupational choice and returns to education.

Family relationships and the transition to college: Coping with loss and grief. At about the same time that students are heading off to college, many of their grandparents and sometimes other older family members are declining in health and dying. This case study shows how the relationships between college students and their families support the students' mental health during the transition to college and how college students can also provide comfort and support across generations.

CHAPTER 20

Maintaining Healthy Boundaries

The relationship between aging parents and adult children becomes even more acute when caregiving issues arise. Many times, the aging parent finds it difficult to accept the adult child's help in the execution of basic living skills (e.g. feeding, using the toilet). It appears to be a fundamental tenet of human nature that we want to be in control of our own lives and do for ourselves, and that this desire persists into the end stage of life. Aging parents may feel burdened, ordered around, and treated in a way they never could have imagined before. In cases in which the adult child had a poor relationship with their aging parent when growing up, the child may begin to find the parent's requests burdensome. Such burdens are more easily identified when the issues such as housing, personal care, will writing, and estate planning are clear.

Communication remains an issue for many families. Adult children and aging parents often struggle with the issue of whether their relationship now is to be that of two adults. Caring and concerned adult children perceive themselves as still being children when they interact with their aging parents. As a result, adult children often make demands of their aging parents that they wouldn't dare make of their in-laws. Often these demands are simply ways to exert power over their aging parents who otherwise have become powerful in society. The elderly may well comply with their adult children's demands, even though they may not desire to do so. They may yield simply because they have grown too tired to fight. If the issue becomes too pressing to ignore, the result may be anger and retaliatory actions by the parent.

CHAPTER 21

Celebrating Milestones and Achievements

Emergent studies are beginning to posit that long-enacted customs and traditions have more imprint on our aging relatives, thus improving their brain health when compared to other activities such as brain games that can be accessed through the internet. Handing to the older significantly improves their overall well-being in terms of cognitive and physical aspects. In a recent study carried out by the Department of Health Aging and Society, University of Victoria, BC, Canada, on empirical evidence between large extended families where relationships are sustained over years through trans-generational communal quarters in India, the results indicated how this eternal space has measurably improved the well-being of these older individuals. Although not entirely age-related, aging mental health may decline with progressing years. Despite the evidence gathered by the Victoria researchers and other similar studies, the findings are normally dismissed as merely anecdotal, even when solid evidence points to the plausibility that simple foundations are the lifeblood of strengthening multifaceted relationships.

Families come together to celebrate events such as birthdays, weddings, christenings, graduations, and anniversaries, as well as preparing for the forthcoming holiday seasons or girding their loins for otherwise daunting activities such as moving house, relocating for a new job, or even the more bittersweet occasions such as attending farewell dinners for loved ones leaving for foreign shores. These "small" or "routine" celebrations bring people in close association with their extended kin and engage even those who are geographically widespread but closely linked through internet and phone communications. Importantly, these significant events serve to bridge the gap to accommodate the older relatives in a space that has disowned them since they had become wrapped and tied in an assortment of handsomely patterned floral print tablecloths.

Cultivating Empathy and Understanding

I wanted to know what we would talk about at this extraordinary meeting, and I decided, somewhat to my own surprise, to start with the first three words of the title: family ties, leaving them off in the first sentence. Few, if any, words cause such immediate and often positive human reactions. Most of us are truly passionate about family. And not just as kids, but as brothers, aunts and uncles, cousins, in-laws, and friends. The family members we imagined at 12 or 18, the one big family, now a timeless echo of Disney in fact. Our own conflicts over shopping for the holidays say just how strong that imagined family is. Our discussion is sure to open with a recognition of the importance of family ties to our well-being.

If we had it in our power to change less than 1 percent of what is wrong in two days, we would indeed become a truly great society. For billions of us, these simple truths seem inconsequential for our everyday behavior. And yet, there is clearly no end to the complex problems we face. So when we are asked what this new phrase means, empathy and understanding, the answer becomes more complicated.

CHAPTER 23

Promoting Intergenerational Activities

There are various ways to allow children to better understand the elderly as well as to build up love and respect for them. Parents, as important role models, should set a good example. Belittling out-of-date habits or mocking speech peculiar to grandparents in front of the children must be avoided. "A wise son makes a glad father, but a foolish son is the grief of his mother," as taught in the Bible. If children see their parents respecting and supporting grandparents, they will naturally learn to do so. Grandparents Day rightly served as an incentive to remember grandparents, but as the occasion of observing it has passed, we should strive every day to promote family ties and to value human relationships, care for the minds and feelings of family members and mentors, listen to the stories they share, and slot in opportunities to interact with senior citizens.

National Grandparents Day, celebrated in September of every year, highlights the value of building intergenerational relationships between youths and senior citizens. Such ties, while underdeveloped in modern society, are critical because, as stated in a 2003 article, "The need for significant ties that are not common to a child's immediate family becomes increasingly important as children develop maturity and individuality." This applies not only to relations with people outside the family but also to members of the older generation within the same family. So, how can families bridge the generation gap and enhance family ties?

CHAPTER 24

Enhancing Family Support Systems

Conflict is not an absolutely necessary phenomenon in human relationships. It is man's quest for conquest that brings about the aggressive tendency to exhibit inefficiency based on interpersonal relationship misfits. At one time or the other, everyone in the world will pass through this institution in life or in death. The American child psychologist and family counselor, John Bradshaw, in his research-based seminar program The Family explained that the problems facing individuals in the world today result from the negative aspects of the function of the family which originally was a mechanism for societal survival. Such must necessarily point to the fact, that the solution to world problems, as it affects individuals resides primarily in the family, the smallest and yet the most important institution of human society. Family is the nucleus, and the first vital point of exploration, it is the instinctual reservoir of meaning and energy in the world-one cannot be without experiencing Family in one breath or the other.

One way of enhancing the family support system is to have a family support meeting. This can be called by anyone in the family (sometimes a member outside the family may also be engaged), and the purpose can be predetermined so that it can be pursued realistically with all sincerity. It can range from how the family should participate in the silent revolution affecting the family such as the child-rearing of adolescent children, to matters about a member of the family who is irresponsible, fluctuating in behavior, and so on. Parent-to-parent understanding is necessary too in these support meetings. Questions like 'what will happen when only one of us has someone to call a family, to plan for? when one of us is geared at achieving an economic feat that is apparently against the norms of the immediate family? and so on, are necessary questions that need to be asked in a family support assembly. Nothing should be hidden for a healthy family and all members need to be prepared for the responsibilities which they automatically are qualified for naturally by their birth in a particular family-the smallest, and yet the strongest institution in the world.

CHAPTER 25

Navigating Intergenerational Conflicts

The word "family" is identified by the study as a "fuzzy set" because of its ambiguous character. A study of the intersection of three fuzzy families, John and Judy Gottman, however, suggests that our genes can all share mechanisms that confer benefits that are not hindered or obscured. To conclude, Nirvana was not a sufficient condition for the practice of the joys of inter-family relationships, but rather the lived Tribal synthesis. While the social fabric of this American family is growing and evolving, it also has deep roots in history. Particularly since this year's award of family advocates, CODA's brotherhood looked as familiar to the ideals of an American family as the author's own nuclear family. If interweaving multiple family identities in one place appears to be very challenging, the reward can be a thick, warm blanket of mutual support. All-important vital structures are flexible, and the ability to think about tensions and contradictions in lives, including family life, in a coherent manner can shape our identities. Regardless of how we interpret these experiences, they keep them meaningful and useful.

When children of elders are expected to participate in the caregiving of their aging parents, other conflicts can arise. In some groups, these demands are the responsibility of the role; in other organizations, these demands pose significant limitations. Consequently, certain forms of caregiving are often labeled burdens or transcend the standard roles of children. These contrasting opinions contribute to intergroup generational disputes related to citizenship performance and caregiving. This essay examines these conflicting intergenerational perspectives and suggests strategies for reducing the conflicts while also increasing our understanding of mainstream and minority group attitudes. Finally, simple actions, the daily habits that become embedded forces of change, are presented here to provide an overview of the small actions that can have an influence on larger.

In some families, parents have difficulty separating from their adult children. Whether it's because of their parenting style or expectations of their offspring favoring dependency, these parents often don't say no to their children. In certain cases, the children strongly resist their parents' efforts to sever the bond. So, the adage that parenting is a lifelong process is occasionally chosen but often assigned. In a culture where children are expected to separate from their marital family once they form their own families, this dynamic is potentially more problematic. This essay encourages and provides steps for assisting families to extricate themselves from generations of entrenched and unproductive behaviors on either end of this common but potentially enabling dynamic.

CHAPTER 26

Embracing Technology in Family Relationships

For the past fifteen years, I have presented programs, workshops, and even consultations to family members struggling with this issue. One of my favorite workshops is "Grandparents: The Glue That Binds Generations." She found that using mutually respected rules of engagement when they are together is essential to strengthen these family relationships in productive forms. Embracing necessary digital technological devices, programs, software, and repair service personnel is a contemporary rule to add to the already established and emerging skills for achieving success while navigating their relationships.

Today's elders can learn much from one another on the use of digital technology to preserve and promote relationships across the generations. My in-laws, Sid and Dorothy Goldman, were in the forefront of older adults in using modern devices to stay connected to family. Concentrated having room on their walls to display photographs of their loved ones, his 93-year-old father asked me to send him only digital photographs. Learning how to use what today is considered archaic equipment, he accessed these images daily. As an alumna of the first class of Brandeis University family therapy master's program, I have incorporated the Goldmans' wisdom in my therapy, workshops, and public speaking focusing on strengthening grandparent-grandchildren relationships.

CHAPTER 27

Preserving Family History and Stories

Heritage is comprised of what we gain through family, society, and national tradition – what we learn from immediate living experiences where we're privy to collective memories of closeness via certain object meanings, stories that convey different life aspects and convey knowledge, aesthetics, and family characteristics – into the treasure we stubbornly keep, making a treasure box that seems to contain more of the past than the future. In recording family history, the possibility of recording a traditional family way of life that complies with the society and its needs seems particularly significant. It's a retrospective that emphasizes the core family and social semantics up until its most reflective sphere – one's own interior, entity of that saturation that reminds us that, in each person, the most enduringly important are biologically and from a social perspective – family and its memories, their wisdom, new meanings that were transformative, and whose purpose wasn't only to grip but to retransform into the community, the family, and its members' compassion.

When people with varied experiences tell their souvenir stories, we find out what lies beneath – story foundations most often stem from family, our roots – our past that continues shaping the present.

It becomes artisans' magic that transforms specific details, feelings, and a whole "picture" recorded in family histories and tradition into an object. The process of completing often seems secondary to sharing stories; however, before we arrive at a story exchange or hearing, there are customs, traditions, knowledge, experiences, history, and heritage preserved in these traditions, regardless of form. Concentration on meanings and ambient context fruition in the youth, appearing passive, but keeping most detail in most often used perceptions – despite or perhaps because of the layering minimalism focus that's marked in their epistemology, making story carriers later emerge within environmental and social ties. Conservation, reinterpretation, and individual transmission of tradition clearly delineate the course of heritage recognition, its preservation, and interpretation – seeing that family empathy and sharing, both personal and belonging towards the general human culture, carries genuine material and spiritual abundance.

CHAPTER 28

Strengthening the Role of Parents

In a world characterized by growing interdependence, it is increasingly important to redefine the conception of social relations in order to preserve the values of cooperation, compassion, and empathy. Reconnecting the world of children with the world of their parents and caregivers—a process heightened by modernity—represents a unique responsibility of present and future generations. There has been a growing trend to focus on the rights of the child at the expense of the rights of the family. To rethink the right of children one must also provide a new definition of family. Equality among family members has been a global priority for some time, but deeper investigation of the concept is needed to allow social and legislative policies to focus on and promote effective measures in that direction. This concept is based on the recognition that despite differences rooted in age, gender, or role, family members are vital to the individual health and the collective development of the human community.

It has long been recognized that one of the most decisive influences that shapes the future of the child is the feeling of security that he or she experiences during the earliest years of life. The parental relationship plays a major role in providing the young child with the sense of security and belonging that is vital for growth. Research confirms the significance of the parent-child relationship in laying a sustainable foundation for the child's future development. When children benefit from an upbringing that is conducive to self-confidence, respect, and independence, the effects are lasting. When children experience disrespect, neglect, or abuse, the effects are likewise long-term, making it much more challenging for them to build healthy relationships, to find meaningful work, and to cope with adversity.

CHAPTER 29

Recognizing the Impact of Family on Well-being

There is a need to recognize the impact of family on individual development. Grandparents, parents, children, and grandchildren speak to the very existence and durability of a family. Therefore, parents, grandparents, and children should have a spiritual bond of love. There is a need for these close relationships to be inculcated in the family members. There is a need to inspire confidence, cheer, encourage, and teach by being role models to the family members. Grandparents should pass their wisdom and experiences to their children, who in turn should pass this wisdom to their children.

As human beings, relationships are so important that without them life would be empty. Just like a bouquet of flowers needs many different colors and types of flowers to be complete, a life without relationships with others would also be empty. The most important relationship people have is with their parents and their extended family who love and care for them. This is because that is where they learn about themselves the most. Elkind maintains that knowing that they are loved gives people security. Without this security, they are helpless. He further asserts that this is because human beings have a strong need for approval and affection from those they love. When they do not get it, they feel rejected and unloved, and their psychological, social, and physical development is often threatened. This is illustrated in many ways. For instance, when a baby does not feel secure, he or she cries and reaches out to be cuddled or held.

Conclusion

Finally, I believe that the impact of labor migration on the health care systems in the host countries is an important issue to be addressed further. A recent article suggested that the EU Commonwealth is in the front line to provide nurses to the UK. Furthermore, data show that between 2003 and 2007 only 50% of the registered nurses came from the EU 2 countries. As the demographic, social, and economic trends currently shape health policies and health care systems in the European Union, I dare to say that the impact of labor migration on the nursing personnel must be of concern for both the Union and the European countries.

Eldercare is not simply a private issue for families to address on their own. It also has a significant impact on the posted workers providing care and on the welfare of the respective home and host countries. According to ILO statistics, the Slovak Republic, Latvia, Portugal, Lithuania, and the Czech Republic rank among the top ten post-Communist EU countries based on the number of posted workers providing care to the elderly. The Slovak Republic and Portugal accounted for 37 and 19 percent of all posted workers, respectively, working in the EU 15 and 18 countries in 2007. With these high percentages of posted workers from the EU 10 and EU 2 countries, one can expect no major implications for the welfare of the elderly in these countries. As noticed, the problem for these countries is rather the massive loss of skilled medical personnel that benefit from job opportunities and higher salaries in Western Europe.